How to Heal Yourself

3 easy steps to Healing, Good Luck, Love
and unlocking the miraculous power within
you to live a healthy, happy and joyful life

Dr. Alexander Khomoutov, Ph.D.

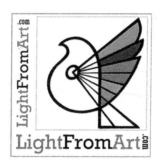

Dr. Alexander Khomoutov, Ph.D.

Get free healing videos and gifts at:

www.LightFromArt.com/healing-gifts

ISBN: 1533581312

ISBN-13: 978-1533581310

How to Heal Yourself

We are in an auspicious time on the planet. It is a time where the essential nature of human consciousness is evolving in profound ways. We are entering into a new reality – one that includes an awareness of our personal spiritual power, and the energetic nature of life. With this change – many people are learning to work with their energy fields to promote healing and wellbeing in unconventional ways. In this book Alexander takes you on a journey, a personal one, where he shares with you what he learned – in his own experience of healing.

In these pages, Alexander shares with you how he discovered not only his "spiritual DNA" but also the power to heal through conscious communication with it! Using kinesiology and other healing practices – he was able to talk to his body and his DNA – and learn innately what was helpful to support him in healing. Although it may sound too mystical to be true – this can be done – and Alexander is one of the pioneers who is using this information in a powerful way for healing and transformation.

Key – Talk To your Body and DNA

Let Alexander's experience inspire you! Every human being has this power - and so do You! The time is now upon us to learn to use it! Enjoy this story of love and healing. May it open a window that allows you to expand what you think is possible – when you dare to dream!

Dr. John G. Ryan, MD
Specialist Medical Doctor, consciousness and energy based healer, University Professor, Author of The Missing Pill, and Harp of the One Heart – Poetic words of Ascension.

Dr. Alexander Khomoutov, Ph.D.

In this book the author shares his personal struggle to heal his own body from unexplained pain.
On his journey he learns a number of techniques that enable him to connect with his Spiritual DNA guidance.

"How to Heal Yourself" will give the readers tremendous insights into how our subconscious mind can be a guiding force leading us down the path of making good positive decisions about our health, happiness, and wellbeing.

Dianne Nassr
An energy healer and contributing author of the book A Juicy, Joyful Life: Inspiration from Women Who Have Found the Sweetness in Every Day.

Dedication

This book is dedicated to my wife Elena and angel Gosha. They inspired me to write this book.

The book is dedicated to all of you who are open to discovering the power within yourselves to live a happy, joyful and healthy life ever after...

Dr. Alexander Khomoutov, Ph.D.

Table of Contents

Acknowledgments

Thank you to my wife Elena. She inspired me to write this book and she was the first reader, who gave me so many suggestions.

I'm so thankful to my parents, who gave me the freedom to do what I love. They always trusted that I would use this freedom in a very positive and loving way. Very special thanks to my mother who showed me how to use the greatest power within. In 1960s and-70s she was already successfully using applied kinesiology – using a pendulum —to determine blood pressure and other things.

I'm very grateful to Lee Carroll and Kryon. Their teachings about the Innate inspired me. They gave me a magic key to unlock the sacred door to my healing and joy.

I'd like to express my very special thanks to Dr. John G. Ryan MD whose book "The Missing Pill" gave me deeper understanding of Spiritual DNA.

I'm so grateful to Dianne Nassr. Dianne taught me how to use Sway test when I was hosting "Healing with Lightworkers" telesummit. This is the main method I use now. She also gave me numerous suggestions to improve the book.

I'm so thankful to Janet Hofstetter for a great copy editing in so tight schedule.

I'm very grateful to you my dear Spiritual DNA for healing, love, joy and happiness. You were so patient to wait so long before I connected to you for the first time ☺.

I'm sending to all of you my Love, Light and Hugs♥.

Alexander Khomoutov

Disclaimer

The author of this book does not dispense medical advice or prescribe the use of any technique as a form of diagnosis or treatment for physical, emotional or medical problems without advice of a physician, either directly or indirectly. The intent of the author is only to offer information of a general nature to help you in your quest for emotional and spiritual well-being.

Please also be informed that any artworks, images, information from this book, etc. are not intended to diagnose, treat, cure or prevent any condition, including: physical, financial or any other problems. The information received through any of these means should not in any way be used as a substitute for advice from a Medical Advisor or other licensed Professionals.

In the event you use any of the information in this book for yourself, the author and the publisher assume no responsibility for your actions.

Dr. Alexander Khomoutov, Ph.D.

Introduction

I had a big moving pain in my chest almost every night for 8 months. It was so strong that I couldn't sleep. I was getting weaker and weaker every day and felt that I was going to die. As you read this book, I'll talk about the sudden death of an angel in our family — our budgie, Gosha — and how that became the turning point in my life and showed me the way to heal myself.

Finally, after 8 months of struggles, I found a very easy solution that worked miraculously for me. And I am sharing my discoveries with you in this book.

1. How it started

Early in 2014, my wife and I were preparing for a 3-week trip to Europe. I was so nervous and busy that I didn't pay attention to the chest pain that I was experiencing at night. I just tried to sleep with it. But just ignoring it didn't help at all. The pain became stronger and stronger. It was a very unusual, moving pain. One day it could be in one place, and the next day in another. Sometimes it moved around my chest and then it might move to my belly. By June, I couldn't sleep at all when I felt it. When I felt the pain in the middle of the night, I reached for a drink of some healing herbal tea with honey and tried to do some work on the computer until the pain stopped. Sometimes it was more than 2 hours before I could fall asleep again. But I kept up my busy schedule. I thought that a 3 km run in the morning, some healing herbal tea and good healthy food would be enough to remedy the

pains I was experiencing. But those things didn't work.

I was regularly sending Good Luck energy, Love and healing hugs to my Facebook community, but I didn't take time to heal myself.

Suddenly, our family's angel, a budgie named Gosha, developed a problem with his eye. He couldn't even open it. I sent him a healing energy and asked my Facebook friends to help him. Many of them sent prayers and healing energy to him, and Gosha's eye healed quite quickly.

But I didn't ask my Facebook friends to help me. And I didn't take the time to heal myself either.

Gosha's eye was healed, but my pains became stronger and stronger. I slept less and less at night, and I became weaker and weaker.

July arrived. Time for our trip to Europe. I experienced pain during the sleepless night before we left for our trip and the next day while doing some final preparations. It continued on the long, sleepless flight to Europe and was still with me throughout that very busy first day.

I went more than 48 hours without sleep. It was a very tough time. The next 3 weeks were exciting, full of interesting events and meetings, but still I was not getting enough sleep. The pains moving in my body woke me up in the night again and again.

Every week I was sending LIGHT & Love and healing energy and Good Luck to thousands of my Facebook friends, but I didn't take time to send Love to myself.

I did not have my usual energy, and this had a detrimental effect on our art sales. That made me anxious and fearful, which made my condition even worse. After 3 weeks of vacation, I returned home exhausted, and my pains became even stronger.

[handwritten margin note: Gosha healed quickly]

2. First attempts to heal myself

When I came back from the trip my health was very poor. My night pain had become chronic and I was 6 kg below my normal weight. I realized I needed to spend time looking after myself. I started a new routine of positive affirmations, exercise, and healthy eating.

I would repeat these positive affirmations out aloud first thing in the morning:

I'm safe

I'm happy

I'm healthy

I'm at ease

And so it is.

I started a routine of running two to three kilometers before breakfast every morning.

I made a special herbal tea with mint, chamomile, Saint-John's-wort, valerian root, ground fennel seeds, Echinacea and honey. I drank some whenever I had some pain and about 1.5 liters during the day between meals. I made sure I ate only healthy foods.

I also started to use a special device that I built myself for energy balancing. It sends electric pulses to acupuncture points.

These healing steps had helped me in the past. But this time, after a week, there was no improvement.

I was scared. I called my family doctor. The secretary asked me about my symptoms and set up an appointment. The next day I got a phone call from the doctor's office recommending that I go directly to the hospital.

I didn't want to go there. I remembered how I had spent a half a day at the hospital waiting in line with bleeding wounds after a bicycle accident. I decided, instead, to seek the help of a professional energy healer.

3. Help from an energy healer

In the middle of August, I decided to find a good energy healer. I love the wonderful book, "Energy Medicine", by Donna Eden [1]. I decided to find a local practitioner who uses Donna's energy healing techniques. On the Internet I found a local practitioner. She had learned from Donna, and was certified by her to perform energy healing. A few days later I had a very helpful 90-minute energy session that helped me a lot. After that session, I had a good night's sleep for the first time in months. I was so happy. But this success was temporary. In a few weeks, the pains came back.

I understood that only by using my inner power could I cure myself. And I have to cure the root of the problem so it won't come back.

Communicate with the Spiritual DNA

4. Experimentation with different healing approaches

From September 2014 to February 2015 I tried many things to heal myself. Sometimes things went well for few days, even a week, but then the night pains would return. Until I found a miraculous cure. Keep reading. You'll find out soon.

4.1 Innate, Spiritual DNA method

Usually scientists talk about DNA from a biochemical point of view without considering the biophysical characteristics. According to esoteric teachings, DNA has also vibrational, quantum nature. Some people call it Quantum DNA, Spiritual DNA, Soul DNA or Innate. Find more about Spiritual DNA at Dr. John Ryan's book "The Missing Pill" [6].

Book

From Lee Carol's channelings of Kryon [2, 3] I found that we can reprogram our DNA for a long, healthy life by communicating with the Spiritual DNA.

So I meditated, connected to my Spiritual DNA and asked

6

to reprogram it to be healthy and balanced to provide a long life with active evolution. In spite of this, the pain came back on some nights. Maybe I wasn't connected properly, when I was doing the reprogramming? I thought. Later in the book you will find out how to check the connection with your Spiritual DNA.

On the 7th of January 2015 I realized that it could be something I had inherited from my father who had similar problems. So I meditated, connected to Spiritual DNA and asked to reprogram my DNA to make me free from inherited problems.

On the 9th of January during my 5 km run, I caught myself thinking about the past and the future but not enjoying the beautiful sunny day right here in the present moment.

I switched my awareness. I felt the fresh air energizing me. I felt joy. Joy shone from inside and out of me, and when I returned I was in the NOW. I got an internal strong message that I didn't need to go anywhere to be joyful. My joy is always inside me and ready to come out, just waiting to be invited to my NOW.

On 11th of January I had the following conversation with my Spiritual DNA. I know that it's hard to believe, but try to be open. I used an applied kinesiology method to communicate to my Spiritual DNA. Read on to find out how.

4.2 Applied Kinesiology (AK) or muscle testing techniques

George J. Goodheart, a chiropractor, pioneered an applied kinesiology technique in 1964 and began teaching it to other chiropractors [4]. While this practice is primarily used by chiropractors, it is also used by other practitioners now, for example in treating allergies [5]. People are sometimes skeptical about whether it will work until they've tried it themselves and see the results. Applied kinesiology, sometimes called a muscle testing technique, is a way to get information from the subconscious.

There are several techniques available. Some methods that you can use to test yourself include:

- Hand Solo Method
- Falling Log Method
- Hole-In-One Method
- Linked Rings Method
- Thumping on Thymus Method
- Pendulum
- Sway Test

I do not describe most of these methods in this book, but you can find out more about them on the internet.

I tried several of these methods over a period of 6 months but I didn't have consistent results with most of them. But I found one method works very well for me – the sway test. I learned it from Dianne Nassr when I was hosting the "Healing with Lightworkers" telesummit [11]. The telesummit was packed with amazing healing information, but this method changed my life. Since that time, I have used only this method because I find it gives me the most reliable results.

4.3 Using the sway test

The sway test is one of the best and simplest methods to get answers from your subconscious mind, Spiritual DNA and Higher Self. It doesn't require the assistance of anyone else. You must be standing to use it (see fig.1), and it takes a bit more time than the other self-testing methods.

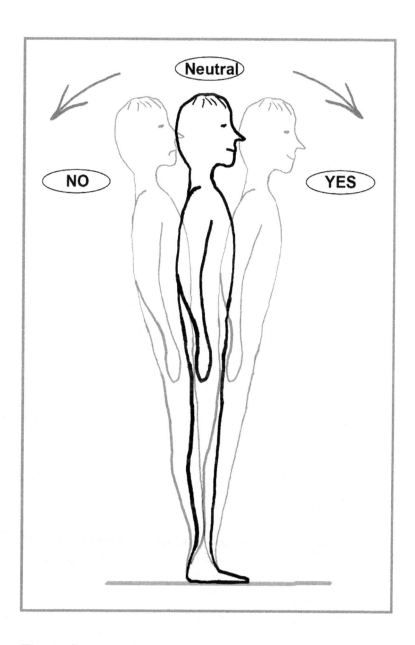

Fig. 1. Sway test.

Preparation

Use the following steps to prepare for the sway test:

1. Go to a quiet room free of distractions, including music and television.

   For me, it works the best when I am alone in the room, but you could do it with somebody else who is willing to do it with you.

2. Stand still, with your feet shoulder width apart for a good balance and your hands at your sides.

   Some descriptions of this method recommend that you face North, but in my experience I find that it works equally well facing in any direction.

3. Let go of all worries and relax your body. If you are comfortable doing so, close your eyes. If you find it difficult to balance with your eyes closed, doing it with open eyes is OK too.

4. Imagine that golden white light beam connects 3 points in your body: the heart, the heart chakra, and the crown chakra. See fig.2.

   This is my own addition to the standard method. If you are just starting to practice the sway method, you could skip this point, but I find that if I do it, I have more consistent results.

5. Use a hand finger gesture while imagining the beam of light (step 4). (This is another one of my additions to the standard method, and it is optional.) Slowly bunch your fingertips together, with tips touching and pointing upward. See fig.3. You could do it with your left or right hand or with both hands at the same time. I prefer to do this with both hands at the same time.

[handwritten margin note: Connect The heart The Heart Chakra and Crown Chakra]

10

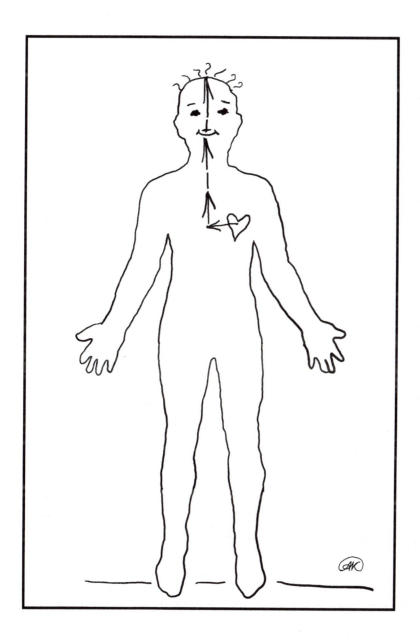

Fig.2. I imagine a golden white light beam connects 3 points: my heart, the heart chakra, and the crown chakra.

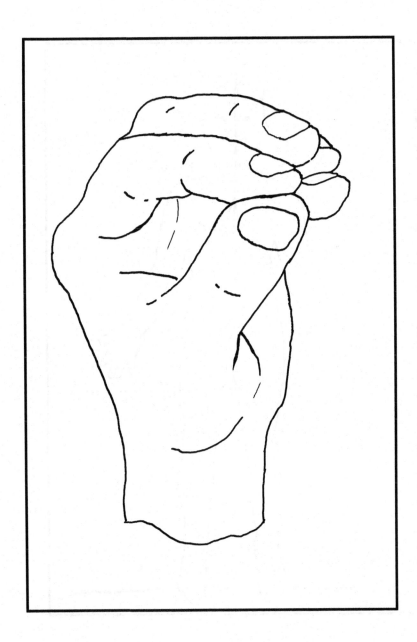

Fig.3. Gesture of balance.

For me, this hand gesture symbolizes connection with Spiritual DNA and balance. I found that with practice I can do just this gesture to establish a connection with my Spiritual DNA almost instantly. If you are just starting to practice the sway method, you could skip it.

Alternatively, you could use another gesture or mudra, for example, the Gyan Mudra, known as the mudra of knowledge. See fig.4. Touch the tip of the thumb to the tip of the index finger, with the other three fingers stretched out. This mudra increases memory power and sharpens the brain. It also enhances concentration and prevents insomnia. Some people also use it as OK gesture. Notice that your body continually shifts its position very slightly in different directions as your muscles work to keep your balance. The movements are subtle, barely noticeable, because they aren't under your conscious control.

Perform the sway test

Perform the sway test using these steps:

1. Make a conscious attempt to communicate with your Spiritual DNA. Say aloud, "I'm connected to my Spiritual DNA."

2. To test that you have a connection, state aloud something that you know that is 100% true, for example, "My name is <your name>". In my case, I say "My name is Alexander".

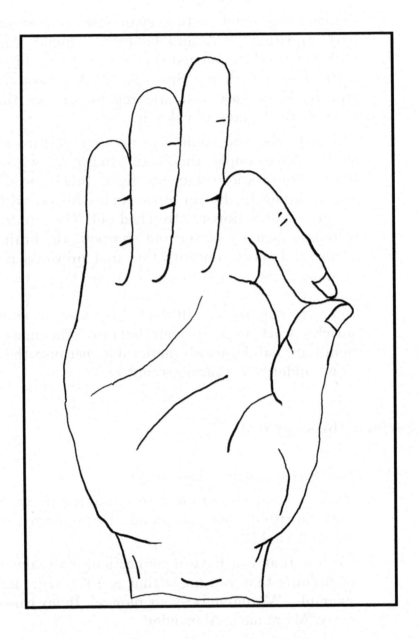

Fig.4. Gyan Mudra – mudra of knowledge.

You are giving your subconscious mind, Spiritual DNA a chance to speak to you in this way. Your subconscious mind, Spiritual DNA knows what is true. When you make a true statement, your body leans forward, because your body is drawn towards positivity and truth. Your body should begin to lean noticeably forward, usually within a few seconds. It means YES.

3. Continue testing the connection with your Spiritual DNA. Make an untrue statement, for an example "my name is <somebody's name>". In my case I say "My name is Elena". As long as you choose a name that isn't yours, your subconscious mind will know that this statement is untrue. Your body will lean backwards within a few seconds. It means NO.

4. Say "Neutral" to have your body come back to the neutral position. I do this between any questions. This is my own addition to the standard method. I find that it makes results more reliable.

5. Repeat the true or false tests described in the previous steps several times in random order to make sure that you are getting reliable results before asking the main question for which you seek an answer.

6. State "I'm connected to my Spiritual DNA". Your body should begin to lean noticeably forward, usually within a few seconds. It means that you are ready to communicate with your Spiritual DNA.

7. Now you are ready to ask your main question. Ask your question in a way that can be answered with just "Yes" or "No." Then if your body leans forward the answer is "Yes," but if it leans backwards then the answer is "No."

Some tips for getting more reliable responses:

- Allow your body to sway on its own. Don't force it. Be patient! Practice every day with questions to which you know the answers already. When you'll have reliable answers then you are ready to ask some other questions. Your body's response time will shorten significantly after you practice every day for several weeks.

- When you ask questions, keep your mind clear of other thoughts. Stay focused on the question you are asking. If your thoughts are wandering, it will be difficult for your subconscious mind, your Spiritual DNA, to determine exactly what you are really asking. What if, for example, after your question you immediately begin thinking about the argument you had with somebody today? You'll probably sway backwards because the memory of that event is negative, and your body will naturally want to move away from it.

- If you are planning to ask many questions or your testing is taking more time than usual, it's a good idea to recheck your baseline periodically. Use a question for which you know the correct answer, for example your name and somebody else's name. If you get the right response, then continue your session.

- Allow love to fill your heart. Do not think about yourself negatively.

- Prepare your questions carefully. The wording of the question has to be exact. Ensure they questions can be answered with "Yes" or "No".

- Be sure that you are hydrated! Drinking a glass of water 15-20 minutes before the session will be very useful.

If for any reason you can't use the sway method, try the other methods listed on page 8. Try them until you find the one that is most suitable and reliable for you *Can do This*

My wife Elena uses her own method. She calls it the Shifting Energy ball method. Elena told me that when she *Ask you Spirit DNA* is feeling tired or lazy or if she needs a quick consultation, she mentally talks to her Spiritual DNA. Often she does it while lying in a bed, sitting or walking. The body position doesn't matter, but it's important to be in an environment that is free of distractions. A strong intention, focus and a trust that information will come from a loving and benevolent Source is very vital. Being relaxed and open-minded is also very important.

Elena says that she senses a dense energy ball in her solar plexus (about 5" wide) as a YES response from her Spiritual DNA. When the answer is NO, she senses the energy cloud in her back at the same level as the solar plexus. The neutral position is somewhere in the middle.

Sometimes she focuses in her mind on the similar test for connection that I do verbally. It goes something like this:

> *Elena: My dear Spiritual DNA, can you hear me?*
> *Spiritual DNA: Yes*
> *Elena: I love you*

After this often Elena senses chills along her spine and in limbs. It's a sign of a reliable connection and loving response from DNA. Then Elena asks her questions and gets answers in the form of the energy ball shifting forward or backward, as described earlier. Often she can sense answers even before finishing her question mentally.

She always ends session with gratitude:

> *Elena: Thank you so much my dear Spiritual DNA. I love you.*

She feels the chilling sensation again as her body responds with a message of love.

> *Elena: I'm disconnecting now.*
> *Spiritual DNA: Yes*

Sometimes Elena skips the disconnection part. She falls asleep and stays in touch with her Spiritual DNA until next session. That's OK, too.

4.4 Conversations with my Spiritual DNA

11th of January.

I initiated connection as described in chapter 4.3. I always test the connection first as the following:

> *Me: I'm connected to my Spiritual DNA.*
> *Spiritual DNA: Yes.*
> *Me: I'm Alexander.*
> *Spiritual DNA: Yes.*
> *Me: Neutral.*
> *Me: I'm <somebody's name, for example Peter>.*
> *Spiritual DNA: No.*

Sometimes I do this test several times to make sure that I am really connected. I always test the connection before any communications, so I'll be skipping the description of the test for the rest of the book.

I had the following conversation with my Spiritual DNA.

> *Me: Dear Spiritual DNA, would you heal me to be free from night pains in my chest in one day?*
> *Spiritual DNA: No.*
> *Me: In 2 days?*
> *Spiritual DNA: Yes.*

12th of January.

At night, I was woken up by pains again. I drank some herbal tea, then used my healing electric pulse device on the 7 acupuncture points. Sometime later the pain decreased and I went to sleep.

13th of January.

I had a good effective sleep (remember that on 11th of January the Spiritual DNA responded, that my pain would be healed in 2 days), and woke up with a healthy and happy face. I had a nice run even though the temperature outside was -18°C.

I find that I am getting a connection to my Spiritual DNA faster and faster every day.

14th of January.

Alkaline Water

My wife Elena found an interesting video about water and asked me to watch it. This reminded me that I have a device that I built myself a long time ago. This electrical device makes Living Water that is alkaline and has powerful healing properties. I decided to ask the Spiritual DNA about the Living Water and about some other things.

I initiated connection and tested it as described in chapter 4.3 and started the following conversation.

> *Me: Is the Living Water good for healing me now?*
> *Spiritual DNA: Yes.*
> *Me: Are the Sea buckthorn berries good for healing me now?*
> *Spiritual DNA: Yes.*
> *Me: Are the frozen green beans from our garden good for healing me now?*
> *Spiritual DNA: Yes.*

21st of January

I initiated connection and tested it as described in chapter 4.3 and started the following conversation.

> *Me: Are black currants with honey good for my break-*
> *fast right now?*
> *Spiritual DNA: No.*
> *Me: Are raspberries with honey good for my breakfast*
> *right now?*
> *Spiritual DNA: No.*
> *Me: Are oranges good for my breakfast right now?*
> *Spiritual DNA: No.*
> *Me: Are sea buckthorn berries good for my breakfast*
> *right now?*
> *Spiritual DNA: Yes.*

I have asked about the sea buckthorn berries before, but I decided to ask again in case something had changed.

5th of February.

I initiated the connection and tested it as described in chapter 4.3 and started the following conversation.

> *Me: Is the EFT calming technique one of the main*
> *turning points to heal my night pains right now?*
> *Spiritual DNA: Yes.*
> *Me: Is a honey massage one of the main turning*
> *points to heal my night pains right now?*
> *Spiritual DNA: No.*
> *Me: Is a regular massage one of the main turning*
> *points to heal my night pains right now?*
> *Spiritual DNA: No.*
> *Me: Are honey and regular massages helpful as an*
> *addition but not as a main turning point to heal my*
> *night pains right now?*
> *Spiritual DNA: Yes.*

Did you notice how important it is to have a carefully crafted question to get an answer you are looking for? Based on the previous conversation, I used EFT (Energy Tapping Technique) for a quick energy boost. Being in a good energetic shape is very important, especially if you find yourself in health challenging situation.

For breakfast I had fermented beans with sour cream. I excluded black currant, oranges, raspberries and sea buckthorn berries. I had 7 components herbal tea with valerian roots several times during the day. At supper I had some cheese and sour cream and herbal tea with valerian roots. I had used a calming EFT before sleep. The result was a nice sleep with no waking during night.

6th of February.

At breakfast I had a cottage cheese with bananas. I had herbal tea with valerian roots several times during the day to heal myself. At lunch I had some fermented beans with sour cream. At supper I had steamed salmon with slightly boiled sprouted mung beans, raw sunflower seeds and tea with valerian roots. I had a calming EFT before sleep. I had a nice sleep again.

10th of February.

It was a fasting day and I had just herbal tea but without valerian roots. At night I was awakened by pains in the chest again. I treated the 7 acupuncture points using my special device for half an hour. After that, I was able to go to sleep.

11th of February.

During my morning run in the park I stopped by the river and spoke to my Spiritual DNA.

I initiated the connection and tested it as described in chapter 4.3 and started the following conversation.

> Me: Can you do all my requests, which I have asked before in comfortable pace?
> Spiritual DNA: Yes.

In the evening I had 2 cups of herbal tea with valerian

root. That night, I woke with chest pains again. I treated the acupuncture points using my special device for half an hour and then went to sleep.

12th of February.

Today I had a sore throat (tonsillitis). I started healing myself with herbal rinses and herbal tea, without medications. I decided to ask my Spiritual DNA to help me.

I initiated connection and tested it as described in chapter 4.3 and started the following conversation.

> *Me: Can you heal my throat in 24 hours?*
> *Spiritual DNA: No.*
> *Me: Can you heal my throat in 2 days?*
> *Spiritual DNA: No.*
> *Me: Can you heal my throat in 4 days?*
> *Spiritual DNA: Yes.*

13th of February.

I was healing my throat with herbal tea and herbal rinses. I also had some consultations with my Spiritual DNA.

I initiated connection and tested it as described in chapter 4.3 and started the following conversation.

> *Me: Can I have a shower today?*
> *Spiritual DNA: No.*
> *Me: Can I have a bath today?*
> *Spiritual DNA: No.*

14th of February.

I was healing my throat with herbal tea and herbal rinses. I contacted with my Spiritual DNA again.

I initiated connection and tested it as described in chapter 4.3 and started the following conversation.

> *Me: Can I have a shower today?*

Spiritual DNA: No.
Me: Can I have a bath today?
Spiritual DNA: No.

15th of February.

I was healing my throat with herbal tea and herbal rinses. I had the same questions as yesterday to my Spiritual DNA and got the same answers.

16th of February.

My throat felt completely healed by the end of day. I had just one question to my Spiritual DNA.

Me: Can I have a shower today?
Spiritual DNA: Yes.

I was very happy. I slept well all night without any pain in the chest.

For most of the days in February I was doing the following things:

- Working to improve our www.LightFromArt.com website. It was a difficult time, because art is the first thing that suffers in a recession. I was worried about it.

- Sending the Good Luck energy to others first.

- Last thing that I was doing if I had some time is to love myself, and for sure it wasn't enough.

If you dont love yourself first - no healing with take place or not stay

♥ Love and Care about Yourself More

5. The message from Gosha: Love yourself first or die

The more often I practiced connecting to my Spiritual DNA, the faster I was able to connect. I always tested the connections as described earlier.

Gosha aww!

During one session I got an unexpected message: our family angel, our budgie, Gosha, was dying. I didn't believe it, but one week later, on February 20th at 2 p.m., he suddenly died peacefully. We were in shock.

Elena saw Gosha's aura sitting on his favorite branch at night. I heard his voice several times, as if he was still at home. We wished him to be reincarnated and come back to us.

In one of my meditations I asked the question:

"Why Did Gosha die?"

Suddenly I realized that he died to give me a strong message that I have to love myself first and care about myself more, otherwise I'll die.

Now I realized that I was in pain for more than 8 months, because I didn't do this. Any powerful healing method will fail if I do not love myself first. So I have to change my bad habits now and then I can bring more love to others.

I took Gosha's strong message to heart. I started to develop a new habit of loving myself first, then sharing my love with others. It sounds easy, but in reality it is a very difficult task, at least it was for me. When you are doing some exciting projects or you are very busy, it is easy to ignore your own needs. Sound familiar? I remembered the preparation for our overseas trip and the sleepless night just before we left. I remembered preparing for important exams.

So I decided to work hard to develop new habits. I also needed to improve my health as the base for the rest of the changes that I needed to make in my life. I felt that I needed some direction.

So I decided to consult with my Spiritual DNA about the food I ate.

I initiated connection and tested it as described in chapter 4.3 and started the following conversation.

> *Me: Is a millet porridge good for me to eat now?*
> *Spiritual DNA: Yes.*

I also asked about the following foods and got the answer YES from my Spiritual DNA: nori, kelp, vermicelli brown rice, brown rice, white rice, popped rice, quinoa, Alaskan Pollack, bus fish, soul fish, broccoli, celery, carrots, carrot juice, olives, cucumbers, pears, peaches, blackberries, sunflower seed, almonds, walnuts, filbert, coconuts, sweet grapes, watermelon, cantaloupe, sweet apples, bananas, oranges, avocados, cauliflower, raisins, prunes, beets, red pepper, strawberries, grape oil, olive oil, rye bread, cabbage, kefir from 3.5% milk, cheese, feta, bakers cheese.

> *Me: Is a buckwheat porridge good for me to eat now?*
> *Spiritual DNA: No.*

I also asked about the following foods and got the answer NO from my Spiritual DNA: butter, meat, borodinskii bread, sour cream, oatmeal, smoked sprats, smoked sturgeon fish, maple walnut ice-cream, potatoes chips, chocolate, coffee, black tea, eggs, salmon, tilapia, cod, chicken, goose, turkey, raspberries, lemons, milk, cream, cottage cheese, tomato juice, black pepper, vinegar, ketchup, garlic, brandy.

I included this list of foods in the Appendix in this book. You can use that list to ask your Spiritual DNA about the foods that are best for you and your family.

> *Me: Are morning and evening runs helpful for me to heal faster?*
> *Spiritual DNA: Yes.*
> *Me: Are Donna Eden's 5 minute energy exercises helpful for me to heal faster?*
> *Spiritual DNA: Yes.*
> *Me: Is honey massage helpful for me to heal faster?*
> *Spiritual DNA: Yes.*

To build a healthy foundation I decided to do the following things every day:

In the morning:

- Positive affirmations (see chapter 2)
- 2-3 km run
- Donna Eden's 5 minute energy exercises [1]
- Drink a healing tea made with 7 herbs

During the day:

- After 45 minutes of work on the computer, take a break of at least 15 minutes. Do something active.

In the evening:

- 2-3 km run
- Honey massage (10 days complete set)
- Go sleep on time. It doesn't matter what time as long as it is the same time every night.

energetic "
painting Opening To
Love"

- Always get enough sleep.

To make my working day more pleasant and productive I decluttered my home office. I also put a special metaphysical energy art painting "Opening to Love" [8] on the wall just in front of my desk. Elena created it to bring a good luck and love energy to the room. Near the front door I had a "Prosperity" art print [9] that Elena created to bring good luck and prosperity. Before the art print was just pinned to the wall, but now I stretched the canvas of the print on a frame and it looks fantastic. Beside me I placed a canvas print from my photograph "Roses for Love" [10], which I created to bring love and good luck. I framed it, too, just for this occasion. So I have surrounded myself with Love, Good Luck and beautiful inspiring art.

Buy print

do

I also cleaned up my 2 white boards. I started to use one of them just for items on how to improve my health and for reminders how to love myself first. My office looks so great now and I have more productive days. Now I have more time to love myself too. The results are amazing since I established my new habits.

From 24th of February until 6th of March.

Honey Massage

I got a honey massage every day, except March 1st. So I got 7 massages. For 8 days I slept well without any pains at night and felt great the next day.

7th and 8th of March.

I was very busy with preparations for International Women's day and didn't love myself enough. I didn't have a honey massage either.

9th of March.

Very early in the morning I had some chest pains again. It was a very powerful reminder, so on the evening on 9th of March I had the 8th healing honey massage and slept well without any pains.

From 10th to 13th of March.

I had a honey massage every day. Each night I slept well without any pains and I felt stronger every day.

24th of March at 12.30 am.

After 2 weeks without any pain in my chest I got strong pain in the heart chakra. So I decided to talk to my Spiritual DNA.

I initiated connection and tested it as described in chapter 4.3 and started the following conversation.

> *Me: Did I have the pain because of the shift to new energies again?*
> *Spiritual DNA: Yes.*
> *Me: Dear Spiritual DNA could you accept new energy now and in the future only at a comfortable pace, so I'll not feel pain?*
> *Spiritual DNA: Yes.*
> *Me: Dear Spiritual DNA, could you clean my body of any old energies?*
> *Spiritual DNA: Yes.*

I felt more comfortable just after the conversation, with some traces of the pain, but not enough to disturb my sleep.

For the next 4 days I felt very good and free from any pain in my chakras.

27th of March.

I felt some pain in the bump on my eyelid. I have had this bump for years without any problems. Some time ago, I visited an eye doctor to check on it. He told me that it was nothing to worry about and I could easily live with it. It could be removed by surgery, but I didn't want to do that at this point.

28th of March.

My left eyelid was swollen and painful. It has swollen to 5 times the size of the bump. I decided to ask my Spiritual DNA for help.

I initiated connection and tested it as described at chapter 4.3 and started the following conversation.

> *Me: Dear Spiritual DNA, could you completely heal my eyelid today?*
> *Spiritual DNA: No.*
> *Me: Can you completely heal my eyelid tomorrow?*
> *Spiritual DNA: Yes.*
> *Me: Will an application of a propolis tincture to the eye lid be useful to heal it?*
> *Spiritual DNA: Yes.*

I applied it at 8.30 am. By the afternoon, the swollen area had decreased to half its size.

The pain had decreased too, but not completely. I decided to apply the propolis tincture again at 1.25 pm.

Then I talked to my Spiritual DNA again.

I initiated connection and tested it as described in chapter 4.3 and started the following conversation.

> *Me: Can you completely remove the bump from my eye lid?*
> *Spiritual DNA: Yes.*
> *Me: Can you do it by tomorrow?*
> *Spiritual DNA: No.*
> *Me: Can you do it in one week?*
> *Spiritual DNA: No.*
> *Me: Can you do it in two weeks?*
> *Spiritual DNA: No.*
> *Me: Can you do it in one month?*
> *Spiritual DNA: Yes.*
> *Me: Please do.*
> *Me: Can you heal any bad things in my body even if I*

don't know about them yet?
Spiritual DNA: Yes.
Me: Please do.

29th of March.

The swollen area on my eyelid disappeared and I was free from all the pain. But the bump on my eyelid looked bigger than usual, and I felt uncomfortable. So I decided to check up with Spiritual DNA again.

I initiated connection and tested it as described in chapter 4.3 and started the following conversation.

> *Me: Is the bump on my eye lid bigger than usual because I asked you to remove it and you are doing it right now?*
> *Spiritual DNA: Yes.*
> *Me: Please do, but heal the bump area first for now.*
> *Spiritual DNA: Yes.*
> *Me: Can you do it today?*
> *Spiritual DNA: No.*
> *Me: Can you do it tomorrow?*
> *Spiritual DNA: Yes.*
> *Me: Please do.*

30th of March.

The bump was healed.

3rd of April.

In the middle of the day I felt some small uncomfortable pain in the chest. So I asked my Spiritual DNA for help.

I initiated connection and tested it as described in chapter 4.3 and started the following conversation.

> *Me: Is the pain related to the shifting of new energies?*
> *Spiritual DNA: Yes.*
> *Me: Can you heal it today?*
> *Spiritual DNA: Yes.*

Me: Please do. You have my permanent permission to do all necessary adjustments to new energies but only at a pace that is comfortable for me. Could you do it for me?
Spiritual DNA: Yes.
Me: Please do.

I felt good after my conversation with my Spiritual DNA.

After that I had a good night's sleep. I felt very good the next day. That day I continued to ask questions about food that was good for me:

I initiated connection and tested it as described in chapter 4.3 and started the following conversation.

Me: Is salmon good for me to eat?
Spiritual DNA: No.

I asked this question before, but I was hoping that something changed and answer would be YES, but again the answer was NO.

I also asked about the following foods and my Spiritual DNA answered YES: three kinds of fish: bass, sole, Alaskan Pollock, and cottage cheese.

I had some strain in my left eye when reading books that day. So I made the following request to my Spiritual DNA. I initiated connection and tested it as described in chapter 4.3 and started the following conversation.

Me: Could you heal my eyes?
Spiritual DNA: Yes.
Me: Could you heal my eyes today?
Spiritual DNA: No.
Me: Could you heal my eyes tomorrow?
Spiritual DNA: Yes.
Me: Please do.

4th of April.

I noticed that I didn't have strain in my eyes after asking my Spiritual DNA to heal it yesterday.

5th of April.

Our Christmas cactus is flowering today! I photographed it and put it on my Facebook page and sent my love to my friends.

I noticed that I sent my love to thousands of my friends, but I forgot to love myself again. I didn't do my morning energy exercises either.

Continue talking to my Spiritual DNA.

I initiated connection and tested it as described in chapter 4.3 and started the following conversation.

> *Me: Is it good for me to drink beer?*
> *Spiritual DNA: No.*
> *Me: Just a little bit?*
> *Spiritual DNA: No.*
> *Me: Is it good for me to drink red wine?*
> *Spiritual DNA: No.*
> *Me: Just a little bit?*
> *Spiritual DNA: No.*
> *Me: Is it good for me to eat ice cream?*
> *Spiritual DNA: No.*

Finally in the evening I found some time to do energy exercises (instead of first thing in the morning).

6th of April.

I had a good night's sleep. I was so happy. Thank you Spiritual DNA! I noticed some small pain in the right side of my chest for few seconds and then again half an hour later.

I initiated connection and tested it as described in chapter 4.3 and started the following conversation.

Me: Could you heal my pain now?
Spiritual DNA: Yes.
Me: Please do.

It was done at once! Miracle! I felt so good. I was so grateful.

Me: Thank you spirit! Could you heal anything in my body that I even don't know about yet?
Spiritual DNA: Yes.
Me: Could you heal it by tomorrow morning?
Spiritual DNA: Yes.
Me: Please do.

I like to eat ice cream, but my Spiritual DNA answered NO. I decided to ask it again. Perhaps something had changed?

Me: Is it good for me to eat ice cream now?
Spiritual DNA: No.
Me: Is it good for me to eat a maple walnut ice cream now?
Spiritual DNA: No.
Me: Is it good for me to eat a goat milk organic ice cream?
Spiritual DNA: Yes.

This was good news for me!

Most days I use my new habits of eating food that is good for my health. I felt better and better every day.

6. At last I feel cured

Finally, I am healthy again! On April 7th, I awoke after a good night's sleep feeling very happy! I looked in the mirror. WOW: my eyes emanate light, my cheeks are rounded, and I look very healthy. I am back to my normal weight. It doesn't matter what I eat, my weight is very stable. Thank you, Spiritual DNA! Finally, I feel completely cured after almost a year!

I went to my computer to send Light and Love to my Facebook friends without first making positive affirmations and doing my energy exercises. I caught myself on it. "Oh, boy, my old habits are still trying to win, but I'm alert and watching now!" I asked my wife to join me.

> *Me: Elena! Let's do affirmations and energy exercises together.*
> *Elena: I am very busy in the garden. I have to finish pruning today.*
> *Me: Gosha sacrificed his life to send us a message that we have to love ourselves first to be able to send more light to other people. Do you want our new baby budgie, Joy, to send the same message again?*
> *Elena: No, but I am busy...*
> *Me: Let's at least do affirmations, then. It only takes*

a minute.
Elena: OK.

Hooray... We did it.

Later in the day...

> *Me: It's already 2.30 pm and we haven't had lunch*
> *yet. Let's do it now.*
> *Elena: I don't want to...*

Elena was busy. So I decided I'd like to love myself and have lunch at the same time.

One hour later:

> *Elena: I was thinking about your words. Let's have*
> *lunch and do the energy exercises now.*
> *Me: Great! I had my lunch already. But I'll do energy*
> *exercises with pleasure.*

And so we did. I felt so refreshed, as always after energy exercises.

And I went with Joy (our budgie) to write about it.

Joy was sitting on my shoulder, inspiring me.

Later, I got a phone call from a gallery. The gallery was closing up and our business relationship was coming to an end. I was very surprised about my reaction to the news. If I had received the same news a few months ago, I would have grieved and been full of anxiety. Instead, I was thankful for the 20 years of good cooperation I had with the gallery. I sincerely wished good luck to the owner. Somehow I felt that it was happening for my highest good and that a new and better source of income would come in the future. It seems my request to my Spiritual DNA to help me let go of fear is working well!

I'm cured, but to stay healthy and to bring more LIGHT to the people I have to love myself first.

6.1 Three easy steps for Healing, Good Luck, Love, Joy and much more...

Three healing steps that I used are the following:

1. Love yourself first

2. Connect to your Spiritual DNA

3. Ask your Spiritual DNA to heal you in a comfortable pace. Be open and trust the process. Be grateful for the outcome.

I also used this technique for other things. I continue to work on the bump on my eye lid, art, joy... You'll find how I have done it in next chapters. I continue to communicate to my Spiritual DNA and Higher Self to enhance my life and stay healthy and happy.

7. Continuing conversations with my Spiritual DNA

In this chapter, I describe some of my conversations with my Spiritual DNA so you can see how I use the conversations to maintain my health and help in everyday life.

8th of April.

I had a good night's sleep. I am so happy!

10th of April.

Elena wanted to sleep. She slept several hours more than usual.

> Me: You slept a long time today. Is there any reason for it?
>
> Elena: It's because of my transition to new energies.
>
> Me: But you woke me up during the night talking loudly and excitedly when you were sleeping. I touched you to calm you. Do you want me to talk to your Spiritual DNA and ask for your effective sleep without any night dreams?
>
> Elena: Yes, let's do it. But I also want to have dreams that could provide some ideas or guidance in the future, and that could come during my night dreams.

Me: I need your permission to do so.
Elena: You have it.

I connected to my Spiritual DNA and spoke loud enough so that Elena could listen to the whole session.

Me: Am I connected to my Spiritual DNA.
Spiritual DNA: Yes.
Me: I'm Alexander.
Spiritual DNA: Yes.
Me: Neutral.
Me: I'm Elena.
Spiritual DNA: No.

I repeated the above test one more time to make sure that I was really connected.

Me: Dear Spiritual DNA, connect to Elena's Spiritual DNA. Do I have a connection?
Elena's Spiritual DNA: Yes.
Me speaking to Elena's DNA: Please make Elena's night's sleep effective and deep. Let her have dreams that provide ideas or guidance, and let her wake up and record them before continuing to sleep. Heal any diseases Elena has now, even those that she isn't aware of.
Elena's Spiritual DNA: Yes.
Me speaking to Elena's DNA: Thank you Spiritual DNA, for connection and help.
Elena's Spiritual DNA: Yes.
Me: I'm disconnected from Elena's Spiritual DNA now.
Elena's Spiritual DNA: Yes

Then I tested that I was really disconnected from Elena's Spiritual DNA.

Me: I am Elena.
My Spiritual DNA: No.
Me: I am Alexander.

My Spiritual DNA: Yes.
Elena: Great but I didn't give you my permission for healing.
Me: You did it yesterday, but we hadn't a chance to talk to your Spiritual DNA about it yet.
Elena: You are right.

14th of April 2015.

Elena sleeps better now thanks to the Spiritual DNA help.

Today I should celebrate that I have had 35 days of restful sleeping, but I had some pain in a heart chakra again when I went to bed. I tried to massage it in bed, and waited for more than an hour hoping that the pain would go away, but without success. Then I woke up and went to my meditation place and had a following conversation with my Spiritual DNA:

I initiated connection and tested it as described in chapter 4.3 and started the following conversation.

> *Me: Do I have a pain in my heart chakra because some old energies are still in my body?*
> *Spiritual DNA: Yes.*
> *Me: Please replace those old energies with new energies in a comfortable pace. Could you do it now?*
> *Spiritual DNA: Yes.*
> *Me: Could you make my sleep comfortable and effective today?*
> *Spiritual DNA: Yes.*
> *Me: Thank you.*

Just after the conversation, the pain started disappearing. In few minutes I went to sleep without pain and had a very good sleep.

> *I said: Ooooooooooooo, Thank you Spiritual DNA.*

15-18th of April.

I had restful nights and joyful days.

19th of April.

In the morning I looked in a mirror and saw my tired face. I looked a little older than before.

I had some uncomfortable sensations in my heart chakra again. So I decided to talk to my Spiritual DNA at the meditation place.

I initiated connection and tested it as described in chapter 4.3 and started the following conversation.

> *Me: Do I have this uncomfortable sensation in my heart chakra because some old energies are still in my body?*
> *Spiritual DNA: Yes.*
> *Me: Could you remove those old energies and replace them with new energies*
> *Spiritual DNA: Yes.*
> *Me: Am I free of old energies right now?*
> *Spiritual DNA: Yes.*
> *Me: Could you make my sleep comfortable and effective tonight?*
> *Spiritual DNA: Yes.*
> *Me: Could you make me feel and look younger.*
> *Spiritual DNA: Yes.*
> *Me: Please do. Thank you.*

Several minutes later after the conversation with Spiritual DNA, my uncomfortable sensations disappeared.

20th of April.

I had very good night's sleep. In the morning I looked refreshed, rested and younger.

I said: Oooooooooooo, Thank you, my Spiritual DNA. I should talk to you more often, not only when something is going wrong.

I felt good, but I decided to talk to Spiritual DNA anyway.

I initiated connection and tested it as described in chapter 4.3 and started the following conversation.

> *Me: Do I have some old energies in my body right now?*
> *Spiritual DNA: Yes.*
> *Me: Could you remove them?*
> *Spiritual DNA: Yes.*
> *Me: Am I free from old energies right now?*
> *Spiritual DNA: No.*
> *Me: Could I be free in few minutes?*
> *Spiritual DNA: Yes.*
> *Me: Could you make my sleep more effective?*
> *Spiritual DNA: Yes.*
> *Me: Could you make me feel and look even younger?*
> *Spiritual DNA: Yes.*
> *Me: Please do. Thank you.*

21st of April

I had very good night's sleep. I initiated connection and tested it as described in chapter 4.3 and started the following conversation.

> *Me: Ooooooooooooo...Thank you Spiritual DNA. I'd like to have a very effective sleep and wake up in the morning looking and feeling younger every day.*
> *Spiritual DNA: Yes.*
> *Me: Please check every day for the presence of old energies in my body and replace them with new energies.*
> *Spiritual DNA: Yes.*
> *Me: Please guide me in writing a book.*
> *Spiritual DNA: Yes.*
> *Me: Please guide me in creating a video about how to choose art to bring positive energy into a home.*
> *Spiritual DNA: Yes.*
> *Me: Guide me to read books faster and faster every*

day.
Spiritual DNA: NO.
Me: Guide me to read books twice as fast in one month.
Spiritual DNA: Yes.
Me: Thank you.

25th of April.

I had some pain in a heart chakra in the middle of the night, so I decided to talk to my Spiritual DNA.

I initiated connection and tested it as described in chapter 4.3 and started the following conversation.

Me: Do I have any old energies in my body?
Spiritual DNA: Yes.
Me: Replace them with new energies.
Spiritual DNA: Yes.
Me: Did I get some old energies from movies?
Spiritual DNA: Yes.
Me: Did I get some old energies from people around me?
Spiritual DNA: Yes.
Me: Did I get some old energies from books?
Spiritual DNA: Yes.
Me: Do I need to remove old energies and replace them with new ones every day?
Spiritual DNA: Yes.
Me: Dear Spiritual DNA, please remove those old energies.
Spiritual DNA: Yes.
Me: Dear Spiritual DNA, could you make all new cells based on templates of cells when I was 7 years younger at a comfortable pace?
Spiritual DNA: Yes.
Me: Please do. Thank you.
Me: Dear Spiritual DNA, could you make all new cells based on templates of cells when I was 8 years

younger at a comfortable pace?
Spiritual DNA: No.
Me: Dear Spiritual DNA, could you make all new
cells based on templates of cells when I was 9 years
younger at a comfortable pace?
Spiritual DNA: No.
Me: Dear Spiritual DNA, could you make all new
cells based on templates of cells when I was 14 years
younger at a comfortable pace?
Spiritual DNA: No.
Me: Thank you.

So it was possible to use only templates that were 7 years younger.

28th of April.

This morning I was waiting for my partner to play a game of tennis. He was late because the car gate to the park was locked and he had to find another way to come to the court. I didn't know about it because I came by bicycle using another entrance. He tried to call me, but I had left my phone at home. After 20 minutes I decided to talk to my Spiritual DNA to find out what to expect...

I initiated the connection and tested it as described at chapter 4.3 and started the following conversation.

Me: Will my tennis partner come 10 minutes later?
Spiritual DNA: No
Me: Will he come in less than 1 minute?
Spiritual DNA: Yes.

In just a few seconds, I saw him coming to the court from an unexpected direction.

29th of April.

Elena had some problems with ants in the garden. They were building nests in the roots of her favorite strawberries. She tried many different environmentally friendly ways to deal with them, all without success. I advised her to speak to the ants through Spiritual DNA. So Elena had connected her Spiritual DNA to the ant queen's Spiritual DNA.

> *Elena: I'm asking you to move out of the strawberries and give you one week to do this.*

During following week she noticed that ants were very busy preparing their new nest under a stone and moved all of their eggs. So finally we'll have strawberries! You probably are thinking that it's not possible, but I am asking you to try it and see.

3rd of May.

I found a used aluminum gazebo for our garden. I made an appointment with the owner to come to his house to disassemble it and move it to my place. I rang the bell but nobody was at home. I called the owner. He told me that he'd come later. He told me to begin disassembling it. I was worried that somebody wanted to use my hands to do some mischief. So I decided to check with my Spiritual DNA.

I initiated connection and tested it as described in chapter 4.3 and started the following conversation.

> *Me: Is he the real owner of the gazebo?*
> *Spiritual DNA: Yes.*

I started disassembling the gazebo and almost finished it before the owner came home. He was the real one!

4th of May.

A lot of dead tree branches were falling down in the garden and it was dangerous. I initiated connection and tested it as described in chapter 4.3 and started the following conversation.

Me: Is it possible to save some dying white ash trees in our garden?
Spiritual DNA: No.
Me: Thank you.

I contacted a special service to remove those trees.

*   *   *

I have consulted with my Spiritual DNA to get advice in many different aspects of my life.

I always ask my Spiritual DNA to give me what I ask in a comfortable pace. I found that it's a very important to remember to ask about it.

Conclusions

I hope this book has given you an inspiration to use the power within you, your Spiritual DNA and Higher Self to have a happy, joyful and prosperous life.

My healing is within me. Instead of fighting against the nature of the universe in order to heal, I asked my Spiritual DNA to heal me.

I became ill because I was so caught up in pursuing goals, achieving, and helping others. I considered myself last.

Now, unconditional self-love increases my energy. The external world mirrors what is within me. I love myself, so there is more love around me too. I give more to others than before.

Any positivity you bring to yourself, you are bringing to all the people around you. Start to love yourself, and this love will help you and everybody else, because we are all connected - we are ONE.

Sending you LIGHT and LOVE ♥☺.

Dr. Alexander Khomoutov

My confessions to you

Now I am cured and feel so good. I sleep well. I enjoy some foods that I couldn't eat before. My weight is very stable and optimal for me. I have had the most joyful year of my life. However, from time to time I catch myself forgetting to love myself first. For example, today I caught myself sending a birthday gift video "Meditation for a good healing sleep" [7] to my three Facebook friends. I was doing it before my positive affirmations and energy exercises. I have to do those exercises before anything else. So, I turned my computer off, did all of my exercises, and then went back to congratulate my Facebook friends..

From time to time, when I was working on some exciting project, including this book, I would catch myself working without any breaks for several hours or working late into the night. So I stopped doing it, reminded myself to love myself first. Love is most powerful healer for me and for all of us. If you love yourself first, then you can spread more love and peace around the world.

Alexander

Appendix: Food list for Spiritual DNA test for you and your family

#	Name	You	1	2	3	4
1.	Herbal tea					
2.	Black tea					
3.	Coffee					
4.	Beer					
5.	Red wine					
6.	White wine					
7.	Brandy					
8.	Chocolate					
9.	Potato chips					
10.	Raw sunflower seeds					
11.	Almonds					
12.	Walnuts					
13.	Filbert					
14.	Peanuts					
15.	Pine nuts					
16.	Milk					

17.	Yogurt					
18.	Kefir					
19.	Cheese					
20.	Cottage cheese					
21.	Coconut cheese					
22.	Sour Cream					
23.	Cream					
24.	Butter					
25.	Feta cheese					
26.	Safflower oil					
27.	Olive oil					
28.	Sunflower oil					
29.	Grapeseed oil					
30.	Salmon					
31.	Tilapia					
32.	Cod					
33.	Pollock					
34.	Bass					
35.	Sole					

36.	Chicken					
37.	Red meat					
38.	Raspberries					
39.	Lemons					
40.	Tomato juice					
41.	Carrot juice					
42.	Grape juice					
43.	Apple juice					
44.	Black pepper					
45.	Red pepper					
46.	Table salt					
47.	Natural sea salt					
48.	White sugar					
49.	Brown sugar					
50.	Honey					
51.	Vinegar					
52.	Ketchup					
53.	Garlic					
54.	Nori					

55.	Kelp					
56.	Brown rice vermicelli					
57.	Brown rice					
58.	White rice					
59.	Black rice					
60.	Red rice					
61.	Wild rice					
62.	Popped rice					
63.	Millet					
64.	Quinoa					
65.	Buckwheat					
66.	Oatmeal					
67.	Broccoli					
68.	Cucumbers					
69.	Tomatoes					
70.	Carrots					
71.	Olives					
72.	Cauliflower					
73.	Cabbage					

74.	Beets					
75.	Peas					
76.	Celery					
77.	Dill					
78.	Avocado					
79.	Pears					
80.	Apples					
81.	Peaches					
82.	Bananas					
83.	Oranges					
84.	Blackberries					
85.	Blueberries					
86.	Honeyberries					
87.	Strawberries					
88.	Red Raspberries					
89.	Yellow Raspberries					
90.	Coconuts					
91.	Grapes					
92.	Raisins					

93.	Prunes					
94.	Watermelon					
95.	Cantaloupe					
96.	Rye bread					
97.	Wheat Bread					
98.	Smoked sprats					
99.	Smoked sturgeon fish					
100.	Haddock					
Add your favorite foods below						
101.						
102.						
103.						
104.						
105.						
106.						

How To Talk To Your Spiritual DNA

Dr. Alexander Khomoutov, Ph.D.

Bibliography and Metaphysical Art

1.   Donna Eden, David Feinstein, Energy Medicine, 2008.

2.   Lee Carol's channeling of Kryon at: https://www.kryon.com/k_freeaudio.html.

3.   Lee Carol, The Recalibration of Humanity: 2013 and Beyond, 2013.

4.   Ph.D. Mark G. Christensen (Author),   D.C., M.B.A. Martin W. Kollasch (Editor), JOB ANALYSIS OF CHIROPRACTIC 2005, ISBN 1-884457-05-3, 208 p. Publisher: NATIONAL BOARD OF CHIROPRACTIC EXAMINERS

5.   Ellen W. Cutler, Winning the War against Immune Disorders & Allergies, 1998, 582 p.

6.   John G. Ryan, The Missing Pill, 2013

7.   Energized for healing guided 2 minutes Meditation for good effective sleep. Video by Alexander Khomoutov at: https://www.youtube.com/watch?v=r1b1JvGiJCM

8.   Opening to Love – metaphysical art print for love and good luck by Elena Khomoutova at: http://lightfromart.com/node/8

9.   Prosperity – metaphysical art print for prosperity and good luck by artist Elena Khomoutova at: http://lightfromart.com/node/12

10. Roses for Love – metaphysical art print for love and good luck by Alexander Khomoutov at: http://lightfromart.com/node/97

11. Leading-edge Healing group sessions, meditations: 16 hours audio downloads at: http://lightfromart.com/node/121

Other resources

Find out about spiritual metaphysical energy art designed to help you in your first conversations with your Spiritual DNA at:

www.LightFromArt.com

Listen to Lee Carol's channeling of Kryon at:

https://www.kryon.com/k_freeaudio.html

Visit Dr. John Ryan's website at:

http://drjohnryan.org

Visit energy healer Dianne Nassr's website at:

http://diannenassr.com/

Check out Dianne Nassr's article in the following book:
A Juicy, Joyful Life: Inspiration from Women Who Have Found the Sweetness in Every Day, by Linda Joy, 2010.

Watch 5 minutes of Donna Eden's energy exercises at:

https://www.youtube.com/watch?v=gffKhttrRw4

Check out spiritual metaphysical energy art prints designed for Good Luck, Love, and Healing at:

http://lightfromart.com/catalog/3

Discover spiritual metaphysical art cards for Good Luck at:

http://lightfromart.com/node/110

Discover Healing with audio group sessions, meditations: 16 hours audio downloads from Healing with Lightworkers telesummit at:

http://lightfromart.com/node/121

Healing Art

It's not just an art - it's a metaphysical energy art tool for Healing, Good Luck, Love and unlocking the miraculous power within you to live a healthy, happy and joyful life. It's created to ease up your connection to your Spiritual (Quantum) DNA for your healing and...

Discover more at:

www.lightfromart.com/node/14

Connect with Alexander

Thank you very much for taking the time to read this book. I'm excited for you to start your path to healing and to live a healthy, happy and joyful life.

If you have any questions, feel free to contact me at:
www.lightfromart.com/contact

You could follow me on Twitter: @_Alex_K

Become a fan and have a fun at:

www.facebook.com/LightFromArt

You can check out my blog for the latest updates here:

www.lightfromart.com/blog

I'm wishing you the best of health, happiness and success!

Sending you LIGHT and LOVE♥☺.

Alexander Khomoutov

About the Author

Dr. Alexander Khomoutov holds a Ph.D. degree in Building Physics. He has a great passion for writing, photography, and healing art. He also enjoys hiking, tennis, skiing and sending Light. His angels: wife Elena and their budgie Joy are inspirations for Alexander's creations. Joy often sneaks into his pockets or even under his shirt and... makes him laugh ☺.

Discover more at:
www.amazon.com/author/alexanderkhomoutov

Get free healing videos and gifts from Alexander at:
www.LightFromArt.com/healing-gifts

Other Books by Dr. Alexander Khomoutov Ph.D.

Baby room decor ideas: How to bring positive energy to your baby for healing, good luck through unique inspirational wall art decorations.

Check it out at:

www.lightfromart.com/node/130

Find more about new books at:

www.lightfromart.com/Dr-AK-books